THE
DREAMER'S
COMPASS

YOUR GUIDE TO BETTER SLEEP
AND A RICHER DREAM LIFE

BY

JOANN GREIG

Disclaimer: This book is for personal development and entertainment only and does not replace professional treatment. Before participating in activities mentioned in the book, it is recommended you seek medical advice if you have pre-existing conditions, sleep disorders, mental health concerns, or take medication. Avoid exercises requiring focus while driving or under the influence of mood-altering substances.

For any inquiries regarding this book, please email:
joann@dreamlifenz.com

Also available as a print on demand book ISBN:978-1-9911924-9-3

For more information see www.wish-books.com

Cover Design by ebooklaunch.com

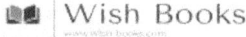 Wish Books

CONTENTS

INTRODUCTION

Welcome to *The Dreamer's Compass: Your Guide to Better Sleep and a Richer Dream Life*. Are you interested in improving your dream recall or managing nightmares? If so, this guide is perfect for you. We'll discuss ways to optimize your sleep environment and habits, remember and record your dreams more effectively, and master techniques to engage with your dream world.

Let us take a moment to consider the impact of good quality and quantity of sleep on life. Too little sleep can have negative effects on daily performance, career pursuits, physical and mental health, relationships, and creativity. On the other hand, restful sleep and imaginative dreams can enhance all of these areas.

Remember, if you are dealing with severe sleep issues, it is worth seeking professional help from a local sleep center or doctor. This book guide aims to help those who wish to dive deeper into the fascinating realm of dreams and improve their overall sleeping experience. So let's get started!

To begin, please fill out the entry quiz at the start of the workbook section. This will be used to track the progress you make throughout your journey.

At the conclusion of each chapter, you will find an example of how some of the key points can be applied in life situations. You will also find reference to relevant worksheets in the second part of the guidebook. You may wish to mark the location of particular worksheets with a Post-it note to find it easily next time. Once you have used up the pages in the workbook, you can switch to using a different journal or folder.

In chapter 7, we review four traditions of working with dreams, including key take-aways from each.

Chapter 8 contains a "cheat sheet": Seven steps for jump-starting your active dreaming.

After you have completed the book, fill out your "after" quiz, and note the areas of improvement.

Your feedback to this email address would be welcome:
joann@dreamlifenz.com

Chapter 1

A Guide to Better Sleep

As we all know, sleep is an essential part of our lives. The quality of our sleep has a profound impact on our daily routine and health. A lack of sleep can cause stress and affect the way we function. In addition, a good night's sleep can mean a rich harvest of dreams to work with later. Therefore, it's crucial to prepare ourselves for a good night's sleep.

Experts recommend that adults get at least seven to eight hours of sleep every night, but the exact amount may vary from person to person. If you struggle to get enough sleep at night, a short nap during the day, up to twenty to thirty minutes, may be beneficial. However, while short naps can be rejuvenating, long or irregular naps may disrupt your sleeping pattern, so avoid napping too close to your bedtime.

We may also choose to establish a bedtime routine that does not involve the use of computers, TV or mobile devices for at least thirty minutes before bedtime. The light from these activities can suppress your body's production of melatonin, which can make it difficult to fall asleep.

Creating a cool, calm, and relaxing environment can also enhance the quality of our sleep. Diffusing essential oils, such as lavender and chamomile, can also improve our sleep quality. Make sure you have good ventilation, so the air in your bedroom is always fresh.

Recording your dreams can help you understand your subconscious better. Keep a dream journal by your bed to record your dreams when you wake up. To improve your dream recall, you can make a dream pillow. Fill a small or large cloth pouch with organic herbs like lavender, chamomile, and mugwort herb to put inside your pillowcase. Make sure the pouch is only used at night when you're ready to sleep. This will turn it into an intimate reminder of your dreams. When you wake up in the morning, inhale the scent of the pillow to jog your memory of any dreams. You could make the pillow even more special by adding designs and symbols such as the moon, a Celtic tree of life, or a favorite animal.

The key to a good night's sleep is preparing yourself for the ultimate relaxation. Your sleep setting should reflect your personal preferences, tailored to help you reach a deep slumber. It is important to create a comfortable and tranquil environment that makes you feel safe and relaxed. After all, your bedroom is your personal sanctuary.

Creating a Sleep Haven

Physical comfort during sleep is of utmost importance. To ensure a night free of discomfort, I recommend using natural cotton or linen sheets, and cotton or silk pillowcases. Layer sheets and blankets to provide enough weight for comfort, but not to overheat. Choose the right mattress and pillow, which should provide adequate support and comfort for your body. Invest in a mattress topper if needed. A good mattress helps keep proper spinal alignment, while a suitable pillow supports your head and neck. To maintain a comfortable temperature, schedule a thermostat or open a window to lower the room temperature. Your bedroom should be cool—60–67°F (15–21°C) for optimal sleep.

It is important for most people to have a dark room without any source of outside light or electronics. Even a small amount of light can disrupt your sleep. To prevent this, consider leaving your phone or computer in another room, or set them to sleep mode at night. The blue light emitted from these devices impacts the brain's ability to fall asleep. You could also invest in blue light filter bulbs or glasses that help to cut out blue light. Additionally, there are apps available that adjust the screen color to avoid the light frequencies that keep us awake. Eye masks, particularly those that apply pressure around the eye sockets rather than directly on the eyes, reduce ambient light in the bedroom, making it easier to fall asleep. You can use blackout curtains, earplugs, or a white noise machine to create a sleep-friendly environment. However, some people do prefer their bedroom to have a night light, and it is a matter of personal preference and what helps you to feel the most relaxed.

Another good idea is to use a sunrise alarm clock. It gradually introduces light similar to sunrise into your bedroom to help you wake up naturally. One can also listen to soothing music or sounds from nature or play white or pink noise to set a neutral sound setting to fall asleep to. It may be best to avoid falling asleep wearing headphones though, as they may disrupt sleep later during the night.

To help us fall asleep more easily, it's vital to clear any clutter and remove any disturbing images from the bedroom. Space clearing is an essential practice to create a harmonious sleep environment, as it helps remove negative energy and promotes relaxation. By decluttering our bedroom, we can eliminate distractions and allow for a more peaceful atmosphere conducive to restful sleep. This process can involve organizing personal belongings, removing unnecessary items, and even rearranging furniture to promote better energy flow. Regularly cleaning and airing out your bedroom also contributes to a fresher, more serene space. Incorporating elements like soothing colors, soft lighting, and calming scents can further enhance the ambiance. By dedicating time to space clearing, you pave the way for a rejuvenated and uninterrupted night's sleep. This leads to improved mental clarity, emotional balance, and overall well-being.

Improving Sleep Quality and Your Sleep Routine

Persistent stress and anxiety can have a detrimental impact on sleep quality. Incorporating stress-management techniques into your daily routine can help alleviate tension and promote restful sleep. Consider practicing deep-breathing exercises, progressive muscle relaxation, yoga, or mindfulness meditation to help manage stress. If necessary, consult a mental health professional to address ongoing anxiety or stress-related concerns.

Breathing exercises are valuable tools for easing the transition into sleep. The 4-7-8 breathing technique, for example, is particularly effective for promoting relaxation. To practice this technique, inhale for four counts, hold your breath for seven counts, and exhale for eight counts. This exercise slows your heart rate and encourages a state of relaxation, allowing you to fall asleep more easily.

Establishing a consistent sleep routine is crucial for achieving restorative sleep. Committing to a regular sleep schedule—going to bed and waking up at the same time every day, including weekends—helps to synchronize our internal body clock, making it easier to fall asleep and wake up feeling refreshed.

Designate an hour for relaxation before bed to help your mind and body unwind. This pre-sleep ritual can include calming activities such as reading, practicing personal hygiene, meditating, or listening to soothing music. Even if you've had a poor night's sleep, try to maintain your regular daytime routine to keep your body's internal clock functioning optimally. Engage in relaxing activities like taking a warm bath, practicing gentle stretches, or enjoying a cup of caffeine-free herbal tea to further enhance your pre-bedtime relaxation.

Upon waking, expose yourself to natural light as soon as possible to help regulate your sleep–wake cycle. Morning sunlight exposure sends a signal to your brain that it's time to wake up, which aids in maintaining a consistent sleep schedule.

Be mindful of habits that may disrupt your sleep. For instance, avoid smoking, as nicotine is a stimulant that can interfere with your ability to fall asleep. Limit your fluid intake in the hours leading up to bedtime to reduce the likelihood of nighttime trips to the bathroom. Furthermore, avoid consuming caffeine and alcohol close to bedtime, as these substances can negatively impact the quality of your sleep.

By prioritizing a consistent sleep routine and eliminating sleep-disrupting habits, you'll be better equipped to enjoy a deep, restorative slumber and wake up feeling refreshed and rejuvenated.

Journey to Tranquillity:
A Story of Bedroom Transformation

Sarah, a young and talented architect living in the bustling city of Auckland, New Zealand, was starting to feel the effects of chronic sleeplessness. She found herself tossing and turning throughout the night with an inability to drift off into a restful sleep.

To match her busy lifestyle, Sarah's bedroom was filled with blueprints, cups of coffee, magazines, and anything else she had yet to put away. Despite its colorful vibrancy and bold designs, it failed to be the calming refuge she needed for a good night's rest.

Knowing something had to be done, Sarah picked up a copy of *The Dreamer's Compass: Your Guide to Better Sleep and a Richer Dream Life*. Reading through it, Sarah discovered the concept of space clearing: the decluttering and harmonizing of a bedroom environment so one can enjoy better sleep. Suddenly inspired, Sarah took the advice to heart.

Over several days, Sarah worked on making improvements to her bedroom. She got rid of all the mess, sorting out and storing away paper scraps and magazines lying around. She even shifted her furniture around to promote positive energy. Colors that were once bright and vibrant were swapped for more earthy shades of blues and grays, while harsh lighting was replaced by soft, cozy bulbs. She cleaned and aired the room more regularly, creating a refreshing ambiance.

The transformation was remarkable, with her bedroom going from an unkempt workspace to a calming sanctuary. On the first night in her new space, Sarah felt incredibly relaxed and fell asleep quickly. When she woke up the next morning, she felt energized and brimming with creativity. Her work improved, and soon sleep was no longer an issue; bedtime became her way of unlocking a more vivid dream life and creative ideas. Updating her environment helped Sarah access a world of undiscovered dreams.

Activities

Complete the Worksheet 1 Self-Care Check-In checklist on getting ready for sleep.

See Worksheet 10: Habit Tracker: What I Do to De-stress.

CHAPTER 2

PREPARING TO DREAM

In order to have a restful sleep and set yourself up for a vivid, meaningful dream experience, it's important to prepare your sleeping space. Starting with the physical environment, avoid any activities that may stimulate your mind before bed, such as social media, emails, or news.

To create a peaceful atmosphere, keep your bedroom reserved for intimacy, relaxation, and sleep. Dim the lights and focus on creating a tranquil environment. You may also consider incorporating the use of crystals into your sleep routine. Crystals have been used throughout history as magnifiers and transmitters and can be particularly beneficial when it comes to promoting restful sleep and vivid dreams.

When selecting a dream crystal, consider clear quartz or other stones like moonstone, selenite, and amethyst. Before using your crystal, be sure to cleanse it with water, smudge it with Sage or other cleansing method. Then, dedicate it to a specific purpose, such as "I dedicate you, dream crystal, to dreams that will allow me to connect with the joy in my life."

For an even more powerful experience, try setting up a crystal grid or a simple altar. For a crystal grid, four rose quartz stones may be placed in the corners of the bed and activated with an affirmation like "I am safe, loved, and protected. It is okay to relax and sleep." An extra grounding element could be added by putting a rainbow obsidian underneath the bed. An alternative can be to lay out a grid on a tray that can be moved to a convenient part of your bedroom.

If space allows for it, an altar can be set up in any corner, on top of a dresser or shelf. All that needs to be there are some objects and figures representing the four elements: Air (East), Fire (South), Water (West), and Earth (North). These could be crystals, shells, flowers, statues of animals or birds, a revered figure, or anything else special that has meaning to you. This helps create a dream-inducing atmosphere. An altar can be as complex or as simple as you wish.

A portable altar can also be created, which can travel with you around your home, outside, or when you're away from home. A jewelry box or carved wooden box containing small objects, crystals, or herbs wrapped in silk cloth should do the trick.

Your Sleep Ritual

Start by going to bed around the same time every night. I like drinking decaffeinated or herbal tea before lying down and avoiding caffeine late in the evening. Incorporate enjoyable habits into your nightly routine; use apps to listen to calming soundscapes, sleep stories, or guided meditations. Diffusing essential oils can make your bedroom feel cozy and comforting for sleep. Natural remedies known as dream aids include vitamin B6, tryptophan, magnesium, zinc, and melatonin precursors—these are found in bananas, tart cherry juice, and nuts; a clinical trial found that taking a combination of melatonin, magnesium, and zinc helped older adults with insomnia get better sleep. However, if you're considering taking supplements as a sleep aid, it's best to discuss this with your physician to ensure there are no contraindications.

Harmony in Crystals:
One Man's Path to Peaceful Slumber

In the serene town of Dunedin, New Zealand, lived a man named Mason, a writer by profession. A master of the written word, Mason had an uncanny ability to weave compelling stories. But in recent times, he had been struggling with writer's block. His creative well seemed to have run dry, leaving him frustrated and uninspired.

Sleep, which was once his sanctuary, had turned into a battleground. His nights were restless, filled with tossing and turning, and his dreams had become hazy and distant. During this struggle, Mason stumbled upon the book *The Dreamer's Compass: Your Guide to Better Sleep and a Richer Dream Life*. Intrigued by the title, he decided to give it a read.

The book suggested keeping the bedroom reserved for sleep, intimacy, and relaxation. It also introduced him to the concept of using crystals for promoting better sleep and more vivid dreams. Feeling desperate and willing to try anything, Mason decided to follow the advice in the book.

Mason began by transforming his bedroom into a serene haven. He dimmed the lights and minimized noise, creating a tranquil environment conducive to sleep. He cleared his room of unnecessary clutter and ensured it was a space dedicated to peace and relaxation. He decided to remove the television that he usually watched before he dropped off to sleep.

He then ventured into the world of crystals. He chose a clear quartz, a moonstone, a selenite, and an amethyst—each stone known for its potential to enhance dreams and promote restful sleep. Mason cleansed each crystal with water and smudged them with Sage, dedicating them to his pursuit of rich dreams and creative inspiration.

Guided by the book, Mason set up a crystal grid around his bed. He placed four rose quartz stones at the corners and a rainbow obsidian underneath the bed for grounding. As he activated the grid, he affirmed, "I am safe, loved, and protected. It is now okay to relax and sleep."

With a spare corner in his room, Mason also set up a small altar. He adorned it with elements representing Air, Fire, Water, and Earth—a feather, a small candle, a seashell he had found at the beach, and a chunk of raw emerald. This, he found, created a dream-inducing atmosphere.

And when Mason had to travel, he carried with him a portable altar, a small carved wooden box containing tiny objects and herbs, wrapped in silk cloth. The dream box altar proved to be a calming and dream-inducing travel companion.

The transformation was profound. Mason began sleeping soundly, and his dreams became vivid and filled with stories waiting to be told.

His writer's block crumbled, and he was back to creating mesmerizing tales. His bedroom had turned into a nurturing cocoon and his dreams a rich source for stories. And in his journey, Mason had found a unique blend of self-care and creativity, all thanks to the wisdom of *The Dreamer's Compass*.

Activities

Complete the Worksheet 2: Self-Care Check-In checklist.

Consider adding these to enhance your dream life.

CHAPTER 3

REMEMBERING YOUR DREAMS

Keeping Track of Your Dreams

A dream journal is an essential tool for self-discovery. It can be one of the most important books that you will ever read, as it's about your life. Whether it's a record of dreams that reflect recurring life themes or reveal purpose and destiny, keeping track of your inner journeys is key to gaining insights into yourself.

However, what makes it so tricky is that dreams are forgotten quickly after REM sleep. Waking up right after this kind of sleep can allow you to recall complete dreams in full detail. But if you wait five minutes, your recollection may only consist of fragments. And at ten minutes after REM sleep, you may have virtually no memory of what happened while you were dreaming. Thus, it's important to jot down as much as possible while it is still fresh in your mind.

You can use any type of journal or notebook for your dream diary. A spiral-bound notebook could be suitable. This way you can divide each page into two sections: on the left side write down all the facts about your dream, such as date and content; on the right side note your feelings, associations, and interpretations. To stimulate recording more dreams, try pre-dating your journal—it sets up an expectation that you will keep track of them! In time, this collection of notes may become your own personal dictionary to learn the meanings behind each dream symbol.

Come up with a name for your dream. Write down important details, such as colors, symbols, and feelings. Drawing what you remember can be helpful as well. Recording your dream is also useful, but make sure to transcribe it later for easy reference. Record as many details as you can. Taking action to honor your dreams is another option—if you have a guardian animal in your dream, for instance, you can show appreciation by eating its favorite food.

What to Write Down

Make a dream dictionary that is unique to you. For example, you can get a binder, labels, and dividers. As you dream, write down each symbol alphabetically or categorically. You can give the symbol a title and date and illustrate it with a drawing. You may also want to include shamanic journeys or special synchronicities from daily life that make you aware that waking life can also be like a dream.

Recording a spoken dream account online can be a convenient approach that lets us search on key words in dreams and dates at a later time.

Another possibility is to draw a tarot card each morning to provide insight into the day's events, and make a note of how these manifest during the day.

Remembering Your Dreams

Remembering your dreams can be simple. Just write them down in your journal or tell yourself before you sleep that you'll remember them. If you're facing an issue, tell yourself that you'll dream about a solution and remember it. Affirmation is the key: "I will recall my dreams, record them, and understand their meaning."

One trick is to drink half a glass of water with the affirmation: "Tonight I remember my dreams." If no dream recall comes, drink the rest of the water saying, "I recall my dreams now and through the day." This often stimulates dream recall. You can also use creative visualization by imagining yourself waking up and writing down your dreams. Feel satisfied because you've recorded your dreams.

If you have trouble recalling dreams, jot down any images or feelings that come to mind. When you wake up, try shifting your body around in different positions, as this may bring back a dream from the night before. Also, it helps to ask yourself questions mentally about the night's dreams and see what answers come up.

Tease apart any dream fragments you can recall too, as they may act as little doorways leading to a deeper understanding of the dream. Additionally, pay attention to the hypnogogic state—the time between waking and sleeping—as it can be a great source of dream impressions and images that can lead to regular or lucid dreaming.

Try replacing any negative self-talk associated with sleep and dreams with affirmations. For example, instead of telling yourself, "I can never recall my dreams," affirm, "I easily recall my dreams" or "I enjoy recalling my dreams." Instead of worrying, "I can never get enough sleep," tell yourself, "Tonight I will enjoy deep, pleasant sleep."

Chronicles of Insight: The Power of a Dream Journal

Maria was a high school teacher who lived in the bustling city of Boston. Loved by her students, she had a knack for making difficult subjects engaging and easy to understand. However, Maria often found herself feeling disconnected from her own life, living on autopilot, and feeling like she was missing a deeper connection with herself.

One day, Maria discovered an intriguing book called *The Dreamer's Compass: A Guide to Better Sleep and a Richer Dream Life*, which recommended keeping a dream journal as a tool for self-discovery. Fascinated by this idea, Maria decided to start keeping a dream journal.

Night after night, Maria would wake up from her dreams and immediately jot down every detail she could remember. At first, it was challenging. Her dreams slipped away like sand through her fingers, but she persisted. She learned to wake up directly after REM sleep, which greatly improved her dream recall.

Maria chose a simple spiral-bound notebook as her dream diary. She divided each page into two sections: on the left side, she noted the factual details of her dreams, such as the date and content, and on the right side, she wrote down her feelings, associations, and interpretations. To encourage herself to record more dreams, she even started pre-dating the pages in her journal.

As the weeks turned into months, Maria began to see patterns and recurring themes in her dreams. She started to understand the symbols that appeared frequently, and their meanings began to unfold. Her dream journal was becoming her personal dream dictionary, a tool to help her to decode messages from her subconscious.

One night, Maria dreamt of standing at a crossroads. She felt a strong pull toward a path surrounded by beautiful wildflowers, but there was a fear holding her back. When she woke up, she recorded her dream and reflected on the symbols and her feelings. She realized the crossroads represented a career choice she had been hesitant about—whether to continue teaching or to pursue her dream of becoming a full-time writer. Then she became aware of a third path that she had noticed at the dream crossroads. The third path was both easy and straight, as well as having some wildflowers growing beside it. This path combined elements of the previous two options.

Maria decided to pursue her dream by writing part-time, while reducing her hours in the classroom, inspired by the paths in her dream. The decision wasn't easy, but her dream journal had given her the clarity and courage she needed. Her dream diary had become a compass, guiding her on a journey of self-discovery, helping her to reconnect with herself and to understand her desires and fears. The experience was transformative, and Maria felt a sense of fulfillment she had never known before.

Activities

See Worksheet 3 on dream affirmations.

On Worksheet 4, make a note of any relaxation techniques you use and how they make you feel.

On Worksheet 5, regarding your ideal sleep routine, write down your perfect evening routine.

See Worksheets 6 and 7 on how to set up your dream journal.

Use Worksheet 8 for your notes and sketches.

Chapter 4

Seeing Nightmares in Perspective

Centuries ago, nightmares were thought to be goblins that attacked sleepers and caused breathlessness. Now, we understand them to be frightening or distressing dreams. Causes of nightmares can vary from stressful events in our past that we weren't able to process as children to unhealthy pressure to conform to the expectations of others, or even post-traumatic stress. In other cases, physical issues such as obstructions in breathing passages could play a role.

It's possible too that our deeper minds are giving us information to protect us in the future. Writing down something from each dream—even the ones that don't make you feel good—can help you recognize messages and alerts your mind is sending. I recently dreamed I was at the dentist, reminding me I needed a checkup.

Rewriting Dreams

Think about going back into your nightmare and playing it through a few times. Change the conditions of the dream so that there is a positive result. This may help to improve the unresolved area of your life that was the cause of the nightmare. For example, in your imagination, bring in a supportive figure—like a power animal, or maybe even a revered figure—to accompany you in this dream world. If you're dealing with a child's nightmare, offer them an imaginary toy like a lightsaber or shield to feel safer during their dreams.

For me, I have a recurring dream where I get lost, which is linked to my poor sense of direction in new places. Whenever this dream comes up, I become aware that I can control the future of it, choosing to reach my desired destination instead. If becoming conscious in the dream isn't working for you, try revisiting it later and making changes to create the ending you want according to how it feels true. That way, you can address whatever source caused this dream in the first place.

Amethyst may be beneficial here as well. Not only does its deep purple color signify the third eye and open us up to spiritual dreaming, but it also has calming and balancing effects on emotions. Place an amethyst under your pillow when sleeping or tape a smaller one onto your forehead.

Recurrent Stress Dreams

If you find yourself struggling with recurrent nightmares or feel like you are under psychic attack, then this guidance can help to stop any further occurrences.

1. Break the Connection

Retrieve any items that may connect you to the attacker, and instruct your personal psychic switchboard to refuse all calls from them.

2. Invoke Spiritual Guardians

Call upon powerful spiritual guardians by names that give you comfort, and trust your animal guardians, too, to shield your boundaries. Let your spiritual allies decide how to best restore balance.

3. Cleanse and Restore Your Energy Field

Take a break to do things that relax and nourish you, such as essential oil therapy, smudging, holding black tourmaline or smokey quartz crystals, or taking a salt bath. Physically spitting out or vomiting toxic energy can be effective for dealing with heavy-duty nightmares.

4. Turn to a Higher Authority

Remember that there are higher forces at work here—those of love and justice—should you wish to refer the case onto them for assistance. Archangel Michael is widely called on in such cases.

Say this aloud: "I have been given this challenge because I am strong enough to resolve it."

If disturbing dreams persist, it is recommended to seek help from a qualified professional, such as a doctor or psychotherapist.

Nightmare to Daydream: Conquering Fears in Dreamland

Liam was a construction worker in Sydney, Australia. A hard worker, he enjoyed his job, but there was one thing that disturbed his peaceful life: a recurring nightmare. In this dream, he would find himself lost in an endless maze of construction sites, unable to find his way out. The dream would always end in panic, with Liam waking up in a cold sweat.

After months of enduring this, Liam decided to take action. He came across a book called *The Dreamer's Compass: A Guide to Better Sleep and a Richer Dream Life* and discovered a technique known as "dream rewriting." Intrigued, he decided to try this approach to resolve his recurring nightmare.

That night, as he found himself lost in the maze again, he remembered the book's advice. He took a deep breath and imagined a kangaroo, his personal power animal, accompanying him in the dream. Equipped with an imaginary map and compass, he felt safer and empowered. Suddenly, the maze didn't seem so intimidating anymore.

On nights when he wasn't able to control his dream, he revisited the nightmare in his waking hours, replaying the dream and imagining a positive outcome. He also placed an amethyst under his pillow, which seemed to create a calming effect and open him up to a more spiritual aspect of dreaming.

After some time, Liam began to notice a change. His nightmares became less frequent, and when they did occur, he was able to navigate the maze with ease, eventually finding his way out.

However, there were still occasions when he would wake up feeling drained, as if under psychic attack. The book provided guidance for this too. He learned to disconnect from the negative energy, invoking spiritual guardians for protection. He called upon his animal guardian, the kangaroo, and spiritual figures he trusted, like Archangel Michael.

To cleanse and restore his energy field, he incorporated self-care practices into his routine. He started using essential oil therapy, held black tourmaline crystals, and took regular salt baths. These practices not only helped him with his dreams but also improved his overall well-being.

Liam's journey was not easy, but he kept reminding himself, "I have been given this challenge because I am strong enough to resolve it." With time and patience, he was able to transform his nightmare into a source of personal growth and self-discovery.

The experience had a profound impact on Liam. It gave him a sense of control over his dreams and, in turn, his life. He learned that with the right tools and mindset, he could navigate any maze, whether in his dreams or real life.

Activities

Keep a record of your dreams. See Worksheets 7 and 8.

Use the Habit Tracker in Worksheet 10 to track at least one thing you do each day to help reduce stress.

CHAPTER 5

EXPLORING THE MAGIC OF ACTIVE DREAMING

Your Dream Adventure

The terms *shamanic journeying*, *active imagination*, and *dream gazing* refer to a similar activity—it's like daydreaming but with more focus. You can access the dream world through your waking consciousness. As you sink deeper into the inner realms, the dream world will start to blend with your daily life. You can use daytime dreaming or dream-gazing techniques to transform your life just as you can change things through dreams at night.

To get started, relax your body and mind; let go of any tension by taking deep breaths in for four or five seconds, pausing for a few seconds, then breathing out for four or five seconds. You can do this either sitting up or lying down; it may help if you cover your eyes with a mask or put a blanket over your shoulders while doing so.

Start simple and invite yourself to daydream for a short time if you haven't been recalling your regular dreams. Not only will this help you learn about the dream world, but it is also a great way to work on difficult situations in your life. Just suggest "regarding the current situation I'm facing, I am now entering a dream," and let your mind wander freely while creating the dream. Observe carefully any symbols and feelings that appear—they might offer insight into how to resolve an issue.

Journey to the Tree Dream Gate

Your journey begins with a visit to an extraordinary tree, bringing to mind the World Tree of shamanic tradition. This is a type of tree that has a special significance for you. It serves as a connection between three worlds: the dark world below through its roots, the middle world through its trunk, and the upper world of the heavens through its branches. Once you've found your unique tree, you can use active imagination to return to it anytime. Take a look at an image online or photography, if you need inspiration.

Directions to the Tree Gate

You may use drumming, either live or recorded, or other meditative music or soundscape. Drumming is traditional, since the frequency of the beats help our brain to shift into gear for the inner journey.

Start your adventure by going to your tree, standing in the location where it stands. You may discover that your animal ally is already waiting for you there. If not, then journeying downward into the Earth through the roots of the tree may be necessary. In this case, you will find yourself traveling through a tunnel, which leads to another landscape. Here, you will meet your animal guardian. Allow your guide to lead you in whichever direction feels right, and let the drum aid you in shifting into another space. Enjoy your dream journey!

You can pose questions to your spirit animal such as "what could I do to improve my health or relationships?" and take note of the response. After spending about ten minutes in the dream, come back to where you started, and write down at least three things from the experience.

Additionally, you can invite your animal companion into other dreams if you feel that you have a need for assistance or protection; for example, if one dreamer needs help, they might call on their Mama Bear guide, while another may rely on a Black Panther's assistance. You can even offer food as a way to welcome your spirit animal by eating the food yourself; carrots could be given to a Rabbit ally, while salmon is good for a Bear and steak is ideal for a Wolf.

Journey to Your Personal Sanctuary

Start your journeys with a visit to your safe place. Shamans and other spiritual explorers often begin and end their travels in an imaginary realm, a sanctuary of sorts.

You can make it however you wish it to be. Some people prefer a more elaborate location, and others feel more comfortable in a minimalistic sanctuary that saves them energy.

Take some time to explore the area. What can you see in your mind's eye? What smells do you recognize? Listen closely. Can you hear birds singing or a babbling brook? What is the temperature like? Maybe it's a location from your past, such as your grandmother's garden or a beach you adored during your teenage years. Maybe it's a cabin in the woods or a futuristic crystal fortress. Some people envision their safe space as located at the base of the Tree of Life.

When something alters in this special place, it is possible that something has shifted in your everyday life. Give the space a good look to see what you can reveal. Perhaps you will uncover items like books that contain useful knowledge or even tools that could assist you on your trips. Many opt to put together a sacred garden in their sanctuary, taking note of the plants and the healing energy they can offer.

You have chosen a spot that feels safe and secure; nothing unwelcome can enter without your permission. Relax with your eyes closed, and take some deep breaths. Visualize the perfect sanctuary, and make use of all of your senses. This can serve as your base for dream reentry or any other imaginary voyages. It can also be used as an area to wind down after a tiring day.

To return after a dream journey, simply say, "Now I'll return to Sanctuary" or just "Sanctuary!" and you will immediately be back there, and from that location you can transition to the waking world. Take some time before leaving and eventually coming back to the here and now.

Sanctuary in the Snow: A Tale of Peace Amidst the Canadian Cold

A rough and tumble hockey player from Ontario, Canada, Lucas lived a life that was anything but peaceful. His days were filled with the sound of skates on ice, the roar of the crowd, and the constant pressure to win. His nights, on the other hand, were restless, filled with broken sleep and nightmares, as if his subconscious was also locked in a brutal hockey game.

In his desperation for respite, Lucas stumbled upon the concept of creating a personal sanctuary through active dreaming in a book called *The Dreamer's Compass: A Guide to Better Sleep and a Richer Dream Life*. Intrigued, he decided to give it a go. He yearned for a place that was calm, quiet, and undisturbed by the competitiveness of his waking life.

Lucas closed his eyes, breathed in deeply, and started envisioning his sanctuary. He took himself back to the serene cottage his family used to visit when he was a child. Nestled in the heart of the Canadian woods, the cottage was surrounded by towering evergreens and sat beside a tranquil, crystal-clear lake.

Lucas could smell the fresh pine in the air and hear the soft rustling of the leaves. He could feel the crisp air against his skin, reminiscent of the cool mornings in the forest. The calm, peaceful surroundings immediately made him feel safe and secure. He imagined a small, warm cabin with a roaring fire, cozy and inviting, completely shielded from the outside world.

As he explored his sanctuary, he came across a little garden filled with healing herbs and flowers, their scents wafting through the air, promoting a sense of calm. He noticed a book on a wooden table and discovered its pages filled with wisdom that could guide him through his inner journeys.

Over time, Lucas made regular visits to his personal sanctuary, using it as a base for his dream journeys and a place to relax after long, tiring days. He discovered that the more he visited this place, the more restful his sleep became, and the nightmares that once haunted him began to fade away.

One night, after a particularly intense hockey game, Lucas found himself in his sanctuary. This time, he noticed a new addition: a small hockey puck, resting on the table beside the book. It was a reminder of his waking life, an indication that his sanctuary was not an escape, but a place to find balance and peace amidst the chaos.

With this realization, Lucas learned to carry the tranquility of his sanctuary into his waking life. His personal sanctuary became his haven of peace, a testament to the power of active dreaming, bringing tranquility to a once restless soul amidst the Canadian landscape.

Activities

Write down at least three things from your dream journeys. You may use Worksheets 7 or 8.

CHAPTER 6

TALKING ABOUT DREAMS

Discussing our dreams can be a powerful tool for growth. Sharing our dreams with others is important, but it's equally important to not overanalyze them; otherwise, we risk losing their primal energy and magic. We should celebrate each other's dreams and support one another in integrating their guidance into our lives. It's crucial that we respect each other's privacy and never presume to know what someone else's dreams (or life) means.

While others can help us draw out feelings and associations from our own experiences, we remain the ultimate experts on our own dreams—much like others are the experts on their own. Dream teacher Robert Moss developed the "lightning dreamwork" method of sharing dreams. It's a technique that encourages the sharing of impactful moments from our dreams, without analyzing or interpreting their meaning.

Let's all continue to express ourselves freely while respecting boundaries.

If you want to share your dream with someone, you may wish to use this method. Or if you like, adapt it to your own purposes in your dream journal.

1. Start by giving the dream a name, and tell the story as simply as possible.

2. The other person should then ask these questions: How did you feel when you woke up? Are there any connections between this dream and something in your life, past, present, or possibly future? What do you want to know about the dream?

3. Invite them to comment on the dream by saying, "If it was my dream, I might think or feel...," not interpreting the dream but expressing their own response to it.

Turning Dreams into Reality

We need to take some kind of action if we want to honor our dreams. This is the best way to bring the energy and inspiration from the dream into our lives. It shows our inner self that we take its messages seriously and are ready to use the inspiration. This could mean researching further a topic in the dream, visiting a location that was in the dream, calling someone who appeared in it but you have not spoken to in a while, scheduling a medical checkup, or even doing an internet search on the topic. Writing down the dream helps us process and integrate the experience better.

Let your dream partner know what actions you plan to take.

Finally, assign a "bumper sticker," a one-line summary of all the themes in the dream.

Throughout history, many writers, artists, scientists, and inventors have been inspired by their dreams and brought forward incredible ideas to benefit society with creativity and technical advances. Consider how you can share your own harvest from dreaming with your community. Have your dreams suggested any projects? Maybe you could express your message through art or literature?

Dreaming Communities

Throughout human history, many communities that have engaged with active dreaming have been successful, even when their environments changed. Dreaming circles can be a great opportunity to work with your dreams and socialize with other dreamers. For example, an Indonesian tribe avoided a tsunami due to their heeding of dream advice, and some people who have paid attention to their dreams have healed serious health conditions before they had symptoms. In other examples, people have avoided travel accidents that they dreamed about by changing their travel plans.

Dreaming groups usually consist of a few members and may offer a sense of community in times of isolation. During and after the Covid-19's lockdowns, meetings started to be held more online. Together we can process our dreams—both during the night and day—with understanding partners who can help us unlock the message behind them and provide support. To make the most out of each session, try to stick to a schedule—weekly or monthly—and keep a dream journal while listening attentively to one another. We should begin every meeting with an intention such as "We come together in the sacred and loving way to honor our dreams" or "We come for healing for ourselves and others."

An interesting challenge for a group is to find ways to involve dreaming in other people's lives. This could be done digitally, through community activities, or with family members. Creatives can express their dreams to the public through artwork or writing. All of these efforts help create a world of dreamers in daily life.

My life coaching business Dream Life New Zealand organizes online dream programs, as well as local events; visit www.dreamlifenz.com for more details, or email me at joann@dreamlifenz.com. Coaching sessions are available to learn about group dreaming and how to experience it alongside our loved ones.

The Dreaming Circles of Brighton: A Tale of Unity and Transformation

In the seaside town of Brighton, England, dreams held a special place in the lives of its residents. Among them was Margaret, a retired literature professor with a fascination for dreams. Margaret believed in the power of dreams to guide, heal, and inspire. She saw dreams as a wellspring of wisdom and creativity that could benefit individuals and communities alike.

Margaret was a follower of Robert Moss's "lightning dreamwork," a method that encourages the sharing of dreams without delving too much into their interpretation by others. She felt a call to create a space where people could share their dreams and gain insights from them, so she decided to start a dreaming circle.

The first meeting took place in Margaret's cozy living room, with its floor-to-ceiling bookshelves and the comforting scent of old books. The group was small, consisting of friends and acquaintances, but the room was filled with anticipation and curiosity.

Margaret began the meeting by explaining the importance of respecting one another's dreams and privacy. She emphasized the value of self-expression and the importance of not overanalyzing dreams to preserve their magic. She then shared the process of "lightning dreamwork" with the group.

In the weeks that followed, the group would gather, share their dreams, discuss feelings and connections, and express their responses without judgment. Each meeting ended with the participants deciding on an action inspired by their dreams, a commitment to honor the wisdom of their dreaming minds.

One of the members, a local artist named James, was inspired by a recurring dream of a beautiful, serene lake surrounded by vibrant flowers. He decided to create a series of paintings based on this dream, which later evolved into a successful exhibition.

The dreaming circle also provided a sense of belonging and connection, especially during the challenging times of Covid-19 lockdowns. The members began meeting online, maintaining the bond they had formed and continuing their exploration of dreams.

Margaret's dreaming circle became a focus of hope and unity in the community. The stories shared and the actions taken helped its members navigate their lives with more clarity and purpose. The circle brought forth the power of dreams, illustrating how they could guide, heal, and inspire not just individuals, but entire communities. The dreamers of Brighton, bound by their shared exploration of the subconscious, became a testament to the transformative power of dreams.

Activities

See Worksheet 9 on Lightning Dreamwork

CHAPTER 7

WORKING AND PLAYING WITH DREAM SYMBOLS

Understanding dream symbols is not always straightforward, as they can communicate through the language of metaphor, imagery, and emotion. Dreams are shaped by our personal experiences, culture, and the archetypal patterns. This subtle dream language calls for a nuanced and multifaceted approach to properly understand them and integrate their messages.

In this chapter, we will journey through the realms of shamanism, Jungian psychology, Gestalt psychology, and Robert Moss's active dreaming, exploring their unique insights into working with dream symbols. Each of these approaches, with their distinct perspectives and methodologies, may provide valuable tools to unlock the messages of our dream symbols. Through their integration, we can cultivate a holistic understanding of our dreams, which offer opportunities for self-discovery and growth.

Shamanism and Dream Symbols

Shamanism, an ancient spiritual practice found in cultures around the world, regards dreams as sacred portals to spiritual wisdom and healing. In shamanic traditions, dreams are not mere subconscious reflections of our waking lives; instead, they are journeys into other realities, places where we can communicate with spirit guides, receive guidance, and engage in soul work.

One key tool in shamanic dream exploration is the practice of shamanic journeying. This involves entering a trance-like state, often aided by rhythmic drumming or other repetitive sounds, to consciously explore the dream realms. During these journeys, dream symbols can be revisited and explored with intention and awareness. This active engagement allows for a deeper understanding of these symbols, as they can be interacted with directly, questions can be asked, and guidance sought.

In shamanic dreamwork, particular attention is paid to power animals and spirit guides. These entities are seen as helpers, teachers, or protectors that can offer wisdom and insight. If such a figure appears in your dream, it is considered a powerful symbol and a gift. They may have a message for you or represent qualities that you need to embody in your waking life.

So, how can shamanic practices be integrated into dreamwork? Here are a few techniques:

1. Shamanic Journeying: Practice journeying to the beat of a drum or other repetitive sound. Set an intention to revisit a dream or engage with a dream symbol. Remember, this should be done in a safe, quiet environment and possibly under the guidance of an experienced practitioner when you're starting.

2. Engage with Your Power Animals and Spirit Guides: If you encounter a power animal or spirit guide in your dream, take time to meditate on this entity. Consider its qualities, its habitat, its behaviors. How might these elements be relevant to you and your life?

3. Dream Incubation: This is a technique where you set an intention before sleeping to receive a dream of guidance. This could be related to a problem you're facing or a question you have. You might ask to encounter a specific dream symbol or spirit guide.

4. Integrating Dream Messages: Make sure to integrate the wisdom or guidance received from your dreams into your waking life. This might involve changing a behavior, adopting new practices, or honoring your spirit guides and power animals in some way.

Shamanic dreamwork provides a powerful lens through which to engage with dream symbols. It invites an active, participatory relationship with our dreams, transforming them into profound spiritual journeys that can offer guidance, healing, and connection with the natural world.

Jungian Psychology and Dream Symbols

Carl Gustav Jung, a Swiss psychiatrist and psychoanalyst, provided groundbreaking insights into the realm of dreams. His theories offered a deeper, more holistic understanding of the human psyche, emphasizing the importance of dreams as a tool for personal growth and self-understanding.

Central to Jung's dream theory is the concept of the collective unconscious, a level of unconscious shared by all humans, holding universal archetypes, symbols, and motifs. These archetypes, such as the Mother, the Hero, or the Shadow, are powerful images and themes that recur in the dreams of people across cultures and eras. They offer a universal language of the subconscious mind, providing deep insight into our human nature and personal psyche.

Jung's dream analysis is closely connected to the process of individuation, a term he used to describe the lifelong journey toward self-realization and wholeness. In this journey, dreams play a pivotal role, guiding us toward integration of our conscious and unconscious aspects, helping us to confront our shadow, and leading us toward self-understanding. Dream symbols are seen as signposts on this journey, shedding light on the parts of our psyche that need attention and integration.

To work with dream symbols from a Jungian perspective, two key techniques may be used:

1. Amplification: This method involves exploring a dream symbol by associating it with similar symbols in mythology, religion, art, and culture. This helps to "amplify" the meaning of the symbol, providing a richer, more nuanced understanding. For instance, if you dream of a snake, you might explore its symbolism in various mythologies, considering how these meanings resonate with your personal experience.

2. Active Imagination: This technique involves entering a dialogue with dream symbols, similar to dream re-entry in the active dreaming approach. In a relaxed state, you allow your conscious mind to interact with the dream symbol, asking it questions, or even engaging with it in an imagined scenario. This can lead to a deeper understanding of the symbol and its significance in your life.

Jungian dreamwork offers a profound and transformative approach to working with dream symbols. It invites us to see our dreams as a bridge between our conscious and unconscious selves, guiding us on our path toward wholeness and self-realization. Through engagement with our dream symbols, we deepen our understanding of ourselves and our place in the world, fostering personal growth and self-understanding. There are many excellent qualified Jungian psychotherapists available who can provide support for clients in connection with dreamwork.

I have included a reference to *The Book of Symbols: Reflections on Archetypal Images* by Archive for Research in Archetypal Symbolism (ARAS). This can help dreamers with amplifying their dream symbols.

Understanding Dream Symbols through Gestalt Psychology

Gestalt psychology, originating in the early twentieth century, is a holistic approach that perceives psychological phenomena as organized, structured wholes rather than the sum of individual parts. Gestalt psychology emphasizes the principle of "Here and Now." It proposes that our current experience, feelings, and thoughts are crucial for understanding our past and future. When applied to dream symbols, this principle encourages us to consider our immediate emotional reactions and associations to these symbols. By focusing on the "Here and Now," we are not just interpreting the symbols based on past experiences, but we are also acknowledging and exploring our present emotional state and how it reflects in our dream imagery.

Another central concept in Gestalt dream work is "unfinished business." Dreams, according to this theory, often represent unresolved issues or unexpressed emotions from our waking life. These unresolved matters manifest in dream symbols, allowing us to address them in a symbolic, nonlinear manner. For instance, a recurring dream symbol may indicate a recurring issue in our lives that requires our attention and resolution.

So, how do we work with dream symbols from a Gestalt perspective? There are several techniques:

1. Dialogue with the Dream Symbol: In this method, you engage in an imagined conversation with the dream symbol. If you dreamed of a roaring lion, for example, you might ask it why it is roaring, what it wants from you, or what it represents in your life. This dialogue technique can provide insight into the symbol's significance in your current life situation.

2. Role-play: This technique involves taking on the role of the dream symbol, embodying it, and speaking or writing from its perspective. This allows you to explore the emotions, desires, and issues that the symbol might represent.

3. Unfinished Business: Identify any unresolved issues or feelings that might be associated with the dream symbol. Reflect on these issues in your waking life and consider how addressing them could impact your dreams.

4. Dream Re-entry: This involves revisiting the dream while awake, either through visualization or guided meditation, allowing you to explore the dream scene and symbols further.

Through these techniques, Gestalt psychology offers us a dynamic, experiential approach to working with dream symbols, emphasizing the exploration of our immediate emotional responses and the resolution of our "unfinished business." By embracing the "Here and Now" within our dream landscapes, we invite deeper self-understanding and personal growth.

Active Dreaming and the Robert Moss Approach

Before we delve into this section, I would like to acknowledge my personal journey with Robert Moss, which has spanned over three decades. I have had the privilege to train closely with him, absorbing his wisdom and teachings, and have completed his Level III dream teacher training. The insights I share in this section are influenced by this personal experience. I cannot do justice to the richness and depth of Robert's teachings in this brief format, but I have included his books for further reading under the Learn More section.

Robert Moss, a master of dream exploration, has pioneered the practice of active dreaming, an original synthesis of modern dreamwork and shamanic methods of journeying to realms beyond physical reality. Active dreaming is not passive; it's about being fully engaged and participatory in our dreams. It brings the energy and insights of the dream world into our everyday lives, transforming our relationship with our dreams from one of bystanders to active participants.

In active dreaming, dream symbols are seen as living entities, portals to other realities, and carriers of energy and guidance. They are not merely metaphors to be interpreted but realities to be engaged with. Engaging with these symbols, we learn to move beyond interpretation to experience, conversation, and action.

Moss offers several practical techniques for this engagement:

1. Dream Re-entry: This is a powerful technique that involves re-entering a dream with a specific purpose. You might want to ask a dream character a question, change the ending of a nightmare, or explore a fascinating dream landscape further. In a relaxed state, you visualize the dream and allow yourself to step back into it, engaging with the dream in an active, conscious way.

2. Dream Tracking: This involves sharing dreams in a group and helping each other to uncover the messages and guidance within them. The role of the group is not to interpret the dream for the dreamer but to offer their insights and reflections, acting as mirrors that can help the dreamer see their dream from new perspectives.

3. Dream Enactment: In this method, you physically act out the dream or dream symbol. This can help embody the energy of the dream, deepen your understanding of it, and reveal new insights.

4. Dream Journaling: Keeping a dream journal is a fundamental practice in active dreaming. It not only helps you remember your dreams but also serves as a place to engage with dream symbols through drawing, writing, and reflection.

Active dreaming invites us to use dream symbols for personal and spiritual growth. They can provide guidance for life decisions, offer healing experiences, catalyze creative inspiration, and facilitate personal transformation. By learning to engage with our dream symbols rather than merely interpret them, we open a dialogue between our conscious and unconscious selves, fostering a deeper understanding of our psyche and enriching our waking lives with the wisdom of our dreams.

Conclusion

Each approach we have explored—shamanism, Jungian psychology, Gestalt psychology, and Robert Moss's active dreaming—offers a unique lens through which to understand and engage with our dream symbols. While they differ in their methodologies and perspectives, they all underscore the profound value of dreamwork for personal growth, healing, and self-understanding.

In integrating these approaches, we can craft a personal dreamwork practice that draws on the strengths of each. We may find the archetypal analysis of Jungian psychology useful in understanding a certain dream symbol, while the active engagement techniques of shamanism and Robert Moss's approach may help us delve deeper into another. It's about finding the methods that resonate most with us and our dream experiences.

Incorporating dreamwork into our daily lives may be as simple as keeping a dream journal, setting an intention before sleep, or taking a few moments each morning to reflect on our dreams. In dream exploration, remember that you are the ultimate authority on your own dreams. While these approaches offer valuable tools and insights, it is your personal experience, and insights that hold the key to understanding your dream symbols and their significance in your life.

A Journey into Jungian Dreamwork

In the coastal town of Nantucket, Amelia, a woman in her forties lived a life that was outwardly simple but inwardly complex. By day, she was a committed librarian, immersing herself in books and stories. But by night, she was a dreamer, a voyager in the realm of the subconscious. For years, Amelia had been fascinated by her dreams, but it was not until she discovered the theories of Carl Gustav Jung that she began to understand their profound significance. She was particularly intrigued by Jung's concept of the collective unconscious and the archetypes within it.

Amelia began journaling her dreams, recording their motifs, characters, and emotions as set out in *The Dreamer's Compass: A Guide to Better Sleep and a Richer Dream Life*. She started to see recurring themes—a powerful, looming shadow, a nurturing mother figure, a heroic quest. She recognized these as universal archetypes, representations of her personal psyche, and the collective unconscious.

In her quest for self-understanding, Amelia used Jung's technique of amplification. One night, she dreamt of a snake coiling around her, its scales glistening in the moonlight. It was not a fearful encounter, but rather one filled with curiosity and wonder. Remembering her dream, Amelia turned to the library, seeking insights from mythology, religion, and art. She found the snake symbolized transformation in various cultures—shedding old skin to reveal a new one. This resonated with her personal feelings of coming to a time of significant change in her life.

Amelia decided to engage with her dream symbol using the technique of active imagination. Sitting in her favorite armchair, she closed her eyes, entered a relaxed state, and reimagined her encounter with the snake. She found herself asking it questions, and to her surprise, it responded. It spoke of her need to let go of past hurts, to shed her old skin of fears and inhibitions. This dialogue revealed to Amelia her deep-seated desire for transformation, indicating the parts of her psyche that needed attention.

Amelia's journey into Jungian dreamwork fostered personal growth and self-realization. Her dreams, once a mystery, had become a compass guiding her toward individuation. In this process, she discovered that the journey is as valuable as the destination, for each dream she navigated brought her closer to understanding.

Activities

Make a note in your dream journal of which dream images or symbols you would like to delve into in, see Worksheets 7 and 8.

CHAPTER 8

SEVEN STEPS TO JUMP-START YOUR ACTIVE DREAMING

This chapter provides a "cheat sheet" that you can use to prompt your dream play.

1. Get motivated: dreams contain valuable messages and experiences for you, so decide to remember your dreams. Your intent counts!

2. Program yourself for dream recall. Of the ways to enhance dream recall, the water technique can work well: Fill up a glass of water and drink half of it before retiring. As you drink, affirm to yourself, "Tonight I remember my dreams." When you wake in the morning, if no dream recall is evident, drink the rest of the water, saying, "My dreams are recalled now and throughout the day." The second half of the water can further stimulate dream recall.

3. Set an intention to dream on a topic you're passionate about, such as one of the following:

    a. Finding your dream job

    b. Finding healing

    c. An adventure in ... (name the dream location)

4. Put an easy flow pen and paper or journal beside the bed to write down your dream as soon as you wake up.

5. Treat each dream like a brilliant gemstone, with each facet containing valuable new insights.

6. After Sleep Dream Recall:

   a. If you can't recall your dreams, try changing position, as sometimes it helps to move back into the position you had when dreaming.

   b. Write down the dream right after it occurs, even if it's a thought, feeling, or word. Give it a title.

   c. Share your dream other others. Talking about it could help you recall more. Remember though, you are the ultimate authority on your own dreams.

7. Honor your dream by taking action: write about it, draw it, speak about it, research information you discovered.

Give thanks for your dreams and enjoy them!

Author's Note and Bio

"Dream weaver, star gazer, and bird whisperer Joann Greig is your guide to a deeper sleep and a richer dream life."

Joann's passion for dreaming started at a young age when she would share her dreams with her mother over breakfast. This love for dreaming followed Joann throughout her career in various fields including social sciences, law, and international relations. She also explored the mystical realms of cultural astronomy and astrology. With over fifteen years of experience in soul recovery and extraction facilitation, Joann's credentials shine brightly with multiple master's degrees.

Joann is an expert in sleep and dreams, and after living abroad for thirty years, she returned to her home country of New Zealand to share her knowledge and experience. She is certified as both an Active Dreaming teacher (Level III) and a Gateway Dreaming coach, and she helps her clients achieve self-understanding and personal growth through transformative techniques.

When she's not working, Joann enjoys exploring local cafes and caring for native birds in a heart-warming rehabilitation project. Joann also wrote, *A Short History of Heaven: Heaven in the Early History of Western Religions and Today*.

Learn more about Joann and embark on a dream coaching journey with her at www.dreamlifenz.com. Her expert guidance is but a click away, ready to illuminate your path to better sleep and a richer dream life.

Your feedback on the contents of this guidebook is welcome addressed to joann@dreamlifenz.com

Please also consider rating and reviewing this book on social media and your online book vendor website. This is much appreciated!

LEARN MORE

Archive for Research in Archetypal Symbolism (ARAS), *The Book of Symbols. Reflections on Archetypal Images*. Taschen, 2010.

Freud, Sigmund. *The Interpretation of Dreams*. Oxford University Press, 1999. Originally published in 1899.

Ingerman, Sandra. *Shamanic Journeying: A Beginner's Guide*. Sounds True, 2004.

Jung, Carl G. *Man and His Symbols*. Doubleday, 1964.

Linn, Denise. *The Hidden Power of Dreams. The Mysterious World of Dreams Revealed*, Hay House Inc, 2009.

Moss, Robert. *The Secret History of Dreaming*. New World Library, 2009; *Conscious Dreaming: A Spiritual Path for Everyone*, Three River Press, 1996; and *Active Dreaming*, New World Library, 2011.

Nauman, Eileen. *Soul Recovery and Extraction: Putting back the Pieces of your Life*, Light Technology Publishing, 2015.

Perls, Fritz. *Gestalt Therapy Verbatim*. Real People Press, 1969.

von Franz, Marie-Louise. *Dreams: A Study of the Dreams of Jung, Descartes, Socrates, and Other Historical Figures*. Shambhala Publications, 1998. Originally published in 1970.

Wesselman, Henry B. *The Journey to the Sacred Garden*. Hay House Inc, 2003.

For further information with healthy sleeping tips: https://www.healthnavigator.org.nz/healthy-living/s/sleep-topics/

Apps can help sleep, for example: the Calm app at www.calm.com

f.lux is a program that adjusts the light generated by your computer, so it is more compatible with natural circadian rhythms.

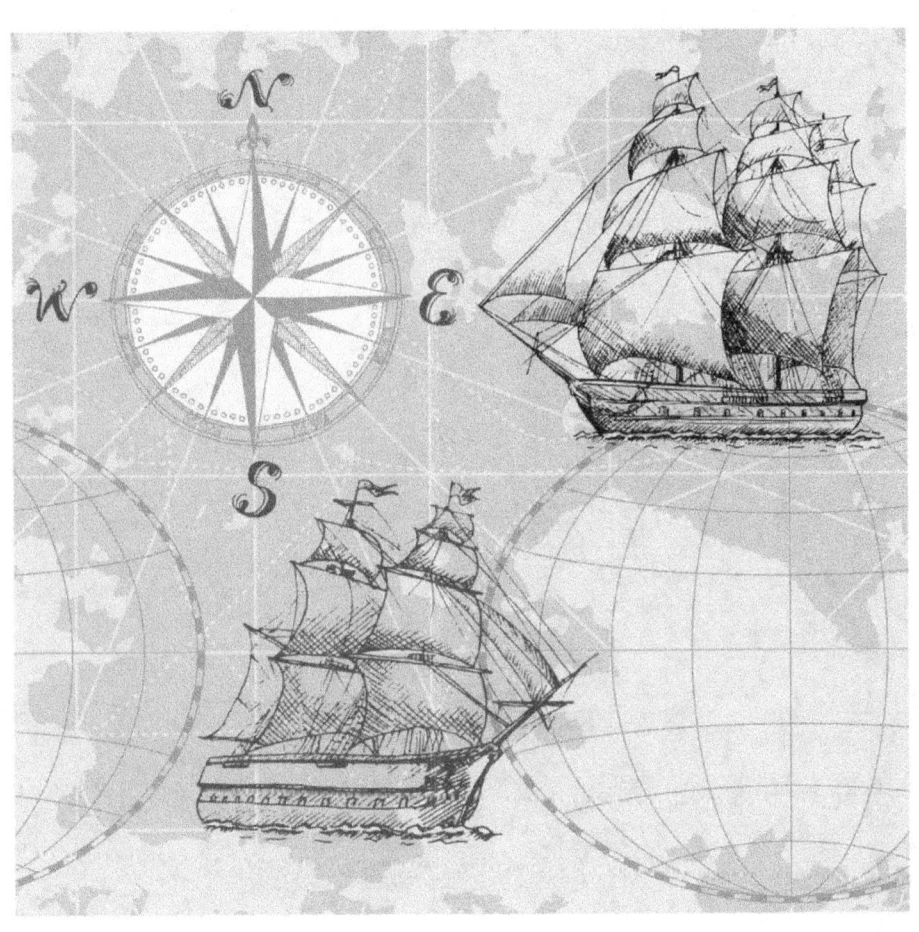

TABLE OF CONTENTS
FOR YOUR WORKBOOK

- Before and After Quiz
- Worksheet 1: Self-Care Check-In—Getting Ready for Sleep
- Worksheet 2: Self-Care Check-In—Consider Adding These to Enhance Your Dream Life
- Worksheet 3: Dream Affirmations
- Worksheet 4: Relaxation and Meditation
- Worksheet 5: Your Ideal Sleep Routine
- Worksheet 6: How to Set Up Your Dream Journal
- Worksheet 7: Your Dream Journal
- Worksheet 8: Your Notes and Sketches
- Worksheet 9: Lightning Dreamwork
- Worksheet 10: Habit Tracker: What I Do to De-stress

BEFORE AND AFTER QUIZ

Before you start working with this guide's exercises, let's see how your sleep and dream life are going. Completing this quiz will help you become more aware of where you'd like to focus and provide a point of reference to assess your growth after completing this book.

Rate how true these statements are to you on a scale from 1 to 10	Pre-rating	Post-rating	Growth
1. I have a good night's sleep most nights			
2. I'm happy with my sleeping environment			
3. My sleep routine helps me relax and get to sleep			
4. I keep a dream journal			
5. I feel positive about my dreams			
6. I remember my dreams frequently			
7. I can tune into my dreams and understand their messages			
8. I can rewrite my dreams if I need to, so that I feel more relaxed with my dreaming			
9. I'm able to share my dreams with others			
10. I know what a dreaming community is.			

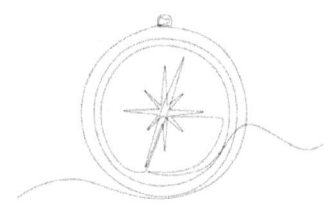

WORKSHEET 1 CHECKLIST

Self-Care Check-In: Getting Ready for Sleep

- [ ] 1. Avoid caffeinated drinks in the evening and late afternoon.

- [ ] 2. Find a quiet spot for meditation, deep breathing.

- [ ] 3. Limit scrolling social media, news, and checking email shortly before bed.

- [ ] 4. Keep to a regular bedtime routine.

- [ ] 5. Dim the lights before retiring to bed.

- [ ] 6. Listen to relaxing music or natural sounds before bed.

- [ ] 7. Keep the temperature in the bedroom pleasantly cool.

- [ ] 8. Avoid eating a large meal shortly before bedtime.

- [ ] 9. Avoid stress by making your bedroom a sanctuary.

- [ ] 10. Avoid electronic and blue light screens before bed.

- [ ] 11. Get sunlight and moderate exercise during the day, but not close to bedtime.

- [ ] 12. Employ clutter-clearing for a calm sleep space.

"Sleep is the best medicine." —Unknown

WORKSHEET 2 CHECKLIST

Self-Care Check-In:
Consider Adding These to Enhance Your Dream Life

☐ 1. Put a dream crystal or crystal grid in the bedroom.

☐ 2. Diffuse calming essential oils.

☐ 3. Prepare your dream journal.

☐ 4. Do a relaxing yoga or stretching routine.

☐ 5. Practice deep, relaxed belly breathing.

☐ 6. Keep a gratitude journal.

☐ 7. Set intentions for your dreaming.

☐ 8. Consider supplements such as vitamin B6 and magnesium.

☐ 9. Enjoy dream-friendly foods, such as bananas, nuts, and tart cherries.

☐ 10. Make a dream altar and/or a mobile dream altar.

☐ 11. What else could you add to this list? Let me know.

☐ 12. Well done!

"Dreams are illustrations from the book your soul is writing about you." —
Marsha Norman

WORKSHEET 3

Dream Affirmations

Instructions: Identify any negative self-talk you may have about your dreams and substitute positive affirmations. See examples below.

NEGATIVE THOUGHT

POSITIVE AFFIRMATION

I can't remember my dreams.	I easily remember my dreams.
I can never get a good night's sleep.	I am loved and it's safe for me to sleep.

"The future belongs to those who believe in the beauty of their dreams." —Eleanor Roosevelt

WORKSHEET 3

Dream Affirmations

Instructions: Identify any negative self-talk you may have about your dreams and substitute positive affirmations.

NEGATIVE THOUGHT   POSITIVE AFFIRMATION

I can't remember my dreams.	I easily remember my dreams.
I can never get a good night's sleep.	I am loved and it's safe for me to sleep.

"The future belongs to those who believe in the beauty of their dreams." —Eleanor Roosevelt

WORKSHEET 3

Dream Affirmations

Instructions: Identify any negative self-talk you may have about your dreams and substitute positive affirmations.

NEGATIVE THOUGHT	POSITIVE AFFIRMATION
I can't remember my dreams.	I easily remember my dreams.
I can never get a good night's sleep.	I am loved and it's safe for me to sleep.

"The future belongs to those who believe in the beauty of their dreams." —Eleanor Roosevelt

WORKSHEET 3

Dream Affirmations

Instructions: Identify any negative self-talk you may have about your dreams and substitute positive affirmations.

NEGATIVE THOUGHT   POSITIVE AFFIRMATION

I can't remember my dreams.	I easily remember my dreams.
I can never get a good night's sleep.	I am loved and it's safe for me to sleep.

"The future belongs to those who believe in the beauty of their dreams." —Eleanor Roosevelt

WORKSHEET 3

Dream Affirmations

Instructions: Identify any negative self-talk you may have about your dreams and substitute positive affirmations.

NEGATIVE THOUGHT	POSITIVE AFFIRMATION
I can't remember my dreams.	I easily remember my dreams.
I can never get a good night's sleep.	I am loved and it's safe for me to sleep.

"The future belongs to those who believe in the beauty of their dreams." —Eleanor Roosevelt

WORKSHEET 3

Dream Affirmations

Instructions: Identify any negative self-talk you may have about your dreams and substitute positive affirmations.

NEGATIVE THOUGHT	POSITIVE AFFIRMATION
I can't remember my dreams.	I easily remember my dreams.
I can never get a good night's sleep.	I am loved and it's safe for me to sleep.

"The future belongs to those who believe in the beauty of their dreams." —Eleanor Roosevelt

WORKSHEET 3

Dream Affirmations

Instructions: Identify any negative self-talk you may have about your dreams and substitute positive affirmations.

NEGATIVE THOUGHT	POSITIVE AFFIRMATION
I can't remember my dreams.	I easily remember my dreams.
I can never get a good night's sleep.	I am loved and it's safe for me to sleep.

"The future belongs to those who believe in the beauty of their dreams." —Eleanor Roosevelt

WORKSHEET 3

Dream Affirmations

Instructions: Identify any negative self-talk you may have about your dreams and substitute positive affirmations.

NEGATIVE THOUGHT	POSITIVE AFFIRMATION
I can't remember my dreams.	I easily remember my dreams.
I can never get a good night's sleep.	I am loved and it's safe for me to sleep.

"The future belongs to those who believe in the beauty of their dreams." —Eleanor Roosevelt

WORKSHEET 3

Dream Affirmations

Instructions: Identify any negative self-talk you may have about your dreams and substitute positive affirmations.

NEGATIVE THOUGHT   POSITIVE AFFIRMATION

I can't remember my dreams.	I easily remember my dreams.
I can never get a good night's sleep.	I am loved and it's safe for me to sleep.

"The future belongs to those who believe in the beauty of their dreams." —Eleanor Roosevelt

WORKSHEET 3

Dream Affirmations

Instructions: Identify any negative self-talk you may have about your dreams and substitute positive affirmations.

NEGATIVE THOUGHT	POSITIVE AFFIRMATION
I can't remember my dreams.	I easily remember my dreams.
I can never get a good night's sleep.	I am loved and it's safe for me to sleep.

"The future belongs to those who believe in the beauty of their dreams." —Eleanor Roosevelt

WORKSHEET 4

Relaxation and Meditation

BEFORE I FELT   AFTER I FELT

Exercise 1 RELAXING MEDITATION

Exercise 2 MINDFULNESS MEDITATION

Exercise 3 OTHER MEDITATIVE ACTIVITY

Note the date and the time you spent in the activity.

WORKSHEET 4

Relaxation and Meditation

BEFORE I FELT   AFTER I FELT

Exercise 1 RELAXING MEDITATION

Exercise 2 MINDFULNESS MEDITATION

Exercise 3 OTHER MEDITATIVE ACTIVITY

Note the date and the time you spent in the activity.

WORKSHEET 4

Relaxation and Meditation

BEFORE I FELT   AFTER I FELT

Exercise 1 RELAXING MEDITATION

Exercise 2 MINDFULNESS MEDITATION

Exercise 3 OTHER MEDITATIVE ACTIVITY

Note the date and the time you spent in the activity.

WORKSHEET 4

Relaxation and Meditation

BEFORE I FELT   AFTER I FELT

Exercise 1 RELAXING MEDITATION

Exercise 2 MINDFULNESS MEDITATION

Exercise 3 OTHER MEDITATIVE ACTIVITY

Note the date and the time you spent in the activity.

WORKSHEET 4

Relaxation and Meditation

BEFORE I FELT   AFTER I FELT

Exercise 1 RELAXING MEDITATION

Exercise 2 MINDFULNESS MEDITATION

Exercise 3 OTHER MEDITATIVE ACTIVITY

Note the date and the time you spent in the activity.

WORKSHEET 4

Relaxation and Meditation

BEFORE I FELT   AFTER I FELT

Exercise 1 RELAXING MEDITATION

Exercise 2 MINDFULNESS MEDITATION

Exercise 3 OTHER MEDITATIVE ACTIVITY

Note the date and the time you spent in the activity.

WORKSHEET 5

Your Ideal Sleep Routine

Instructions: Imagined in sensory detail your perfect evening routine. How would you feel, what you would you wear, who would you be with, and where would you be? What would you do, and where? Write it down below.

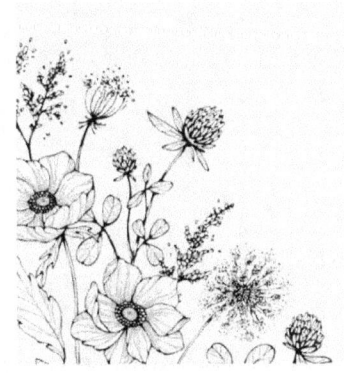

WORKSHEET 5

Your Ideal Sleep Routine

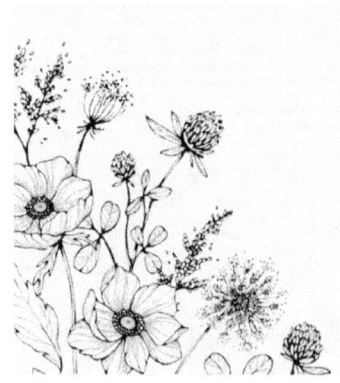

WORKSHEET 5

Your Ideal Sleep Routine

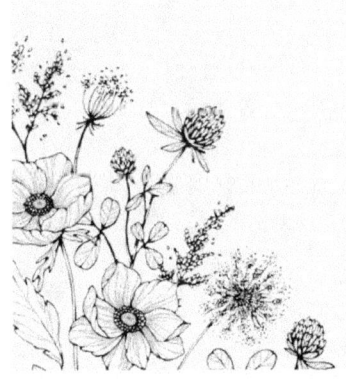

WORKSHEET 5

Your Ideal Sleep Routine

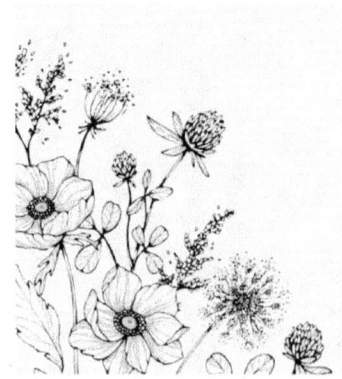

WORKSHEET 6

How to Set Up Your Dream Journal

Instructions: Use these templates to start your dream journal and dream dictionary of symbols, or use your own journal or other format.

Dream #1

DREAM STORY AND IMAGES	FEELINGS AND ASSOCIATIONS
Date:	
Time:	
Place:	
Write down everything you recall, even if it doesn't seem to be a dream. You may include hypnogogic images. You may also wish to include meaningful coincidences, synchronicities, from daily life.	

WORKSHEET 7

Your Dream Journal

Dream

DREAM STORY AND IMAGES	FEELINGS AND ASSOCIATIONS
Date: Time: Place:	

WORKSHEET 7

Your Dream Journal

DREAM STORY AND IMAGES	FEELINGS AND ASSOCIATIONS
Date: Time: Place:	

WORKSHEET 7

Your Dream Journal

Dream

DREAM STORY AND IMAGES	FEELINGS AND ASSOCIATIONS
Date: Time: Place:	

WORKSHEET 7

Your Dream Journal

Dream

DREAM STORY AND IMAGES	FEELINGS AND ASSOCIATIONS
Date: Time: Place:	

WORKSHEET 7

Your Dream Journal

Dream

DREAM STORY AND IMAGES	FEELINGS AND ASSOCIATIONS
Date: Time: Place:	

WORKSHEET 7

Your Dream Journal

Dream

DREAM STORY AND IMAGES	FEELINGS AND ASSOCIATIONS
Date: Time: Place:	

WORKSHEET 7

Your Dream Journal

Dream

DREAM STORY AND IMAGES	FEELINGS AND ASSOCIATIONS
Date:	
Time:	
Place:	

WORKSHEET 7

Your Dream Journal

Dream

DREAM STORY AND IMAGES	FEELINGS AND ASSOCIATIONS
Date: Time: Place:	

WORKSHEET 7

Your Dream Journal

Dream

DREAM STORY AND IMAGES	FEELINGS AND ASSOCIATIONS
Date: Time: Place:	

WORKSHEET 7

Your Dream Journal

Dream #

DREAM STORY AND IMAGES	FEELINGS AND ASSOCIATIONS
Date: Time: Place:	

WORKSHEET 7

Your Dream Journal

Dream

DREAM STORY AND IMAGES	FEELINGS AND ASSOCIATIONS
Date: Time: Place:	

WORKSHEET 7

Your Dream Journal

Dream

DREAM STORY AND IMAGES	FEELINGS AND ASSOCIATIONS
Date: Time: Place:	

WORKSHEET 7

Your Dream Journal

Dream

DREAM STORY AND IMAGES	FEELINGS AND ASSOCIATIONS
Date: Time: Place:	

WORKSHEET 7

Your Dream Journal

Dream

DREAM STORY AND IMAGES	FEELINGS AND ASSOCIATIONS
Date: Time: Place:	

WORKSHEET 7

Your Dream Journal

Dream

DREAM STORY AND IMAGES	FEELINGS AND ASSOCIATIONS
Date:	
Time:	
Place:	

WORKSHEET 7

Your Dream Journal

Dream

DREAM STORY AND IMAGES	FEELINGS AND ASSOCIATIONS
Date: Time: Place:	

WORKSHEET 7

Your Dream Journal

Dream

DREAM STORY AND IMAGES	FEELINGS AND ASSOCIATIONS
Date: Time: Place:	

WORKSHEET 7

Your Dream Journal

Dream

DREAM STORY AND IMAGES	FEELINGS AND ASSOCIATIONS
Date: Time: Place:	

WORKSHEET 7

Your Dream Journal

Dream

DREAM STORY AND IMAGES	FEELINGS AND ASSOCIATIONS
Date: Time: Place:	

WORKSHEET 7

Your Dream Journal

Dream

DREAM STORY AND IMAGES	FEELINGS AND ASSOCIATIONS
Date: Time: Place:	

WORKSHEET 7

Your Dream Journal

Dream

DREAM STORY AND IMAGES	FEELINGS AND ASSOCIATIONS
Date:	
Time:	
Place:	

WORKSHEET 7

Your Dream Journal

Dream

DREAM STORY AND IMAGES	FEELINGS AND ASSOCIATIONS
Date: Time: Place:	

WORKSHEET 7

Your Dream Journal

Dream

DREAM STORY AND IMAGES	FEELINGS AND ASSOCIATIONS
Date: Time: Place:	

WORKSHEET 7

Your Dream Journal

Dream

DREAM STORY AND IMAGES	FEELINGS AND ASSOCIATIONS
Date: Time: Place:	

WORKSHEET 7

Your Dream Journal

Dream

DREAM STORY AND IMAGES	FEELINGS AND ASSOCIATIONS
Date: Time: Place:	

WORKSHEET 7

Your Dream Journal

Dream #

DREAM STORY AND IMAGES	FEELINGS AND ASSOCIATIONS
Date: Time: Place:	

WORKSHEET 7

Your Dream Journal

Dream

DREAM STORY AND IMAGES	FEELINGS AND ASSOCIATIONS
Date: Time: Place:	

WORKSHEET 7

Your Dream Journal

Dream

DREAM STORY AND IMAGES	FEELINGS AND ASSOCIATIONS
Date:	
Time:	
Place:	

WORKSHEET 7

Your Dream Journal

Dream

DREAM STORY AND IMAGES	FEELINGS AND ASSOCIATIONS
Date: Time: Place:	

WORKSHEET 7

Your Dream Journal

Dream

DREAM STORY AND IMAGES	FEELINGS AND ASSOCIATIONS
Date: Time: Place:	

WORKSHEET 8

Your Notes and Sketches

WORKSHEET 9

Lightning Dreamwork

INSTRUCTIONS: Use the Lightning Dreamwork* framework to share dreams with others.

STEP 1: Explain your dream as clearly and simply as possible. Give it a title.

STEP 2: How did you feel upon awakening?

STEP 3: Reality check: Do you recognize anything from your life now or possibly in the future?

STEP 4: Your partner plays the "If it was my dream" game and shares their ideas, thoughts, and feelings about the dream, as if it had been theirs.

STEP 5: Summarize the dream in a pithy phrase, like a bumper sticker.

STEP 6: Identify what action steps you intend to take to honor your dream.

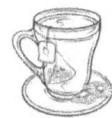 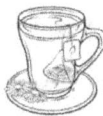

* Based on the work of Robert Moss.

WORKSHEET 9

Lightning Dreamwork

INSTRUCTIONS: Use the Lightning Dreamwork* framework to share dreams with others.

STEP 1: Explain your dream as clearly and simply as possible. Give it a title.

STEP 2: How did you feel upon awakening?

STEP 3: Reality check: Do you recognize anything from your life now or possibly in the future?

STEP 4: Your partner plays the "If it was my dream" game and shares their ideas, thoughts, and feelings about the dream, as if it had been theirs.

STEP 5: Summarize the dream in a pithy phrase, like a bumper sticker.

STEP 6: Identify what action steps you intend to take to honor your dream.

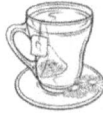 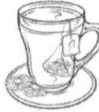

* Based on the work of Robert Moss.

WORKSHEET 9

Lightning Dreamwork

INSTRUCTIONS: Use the Lightning Dreamwork* framework to share dreams with others.

STEP 1: Explain your dream as clearly and simply as possible. Give it a title.

STEP 2: How did you feel upon awakening?

STEP 3: Reality check: Do you recognize anything from your life now or possibly in the future?

STEP 4: Your partner plays the "If it was my dream" game and shares their ideas, thoughts, and feelings about the dream, as if it had been theirs.

STEP 5: Summarize the dream in a pithy phrase, like a bumper sticker.

STEP 6: Identify what action steps you intend to take to honor your dream.

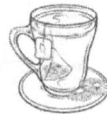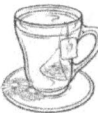

* Based on the work of Robert Moss.

WORKSHEET 9

Lightning Dreamwork

INSTRUCTIONS: Use the Lightning Dreamwork* framework to share dreams with others.

STEP 1: Explain your dream as clearly and simply as possible. Give it a title.

STEP 2: How did you feel upon awakening?

STEP 3: Reality check: Do you recognize anything from your life now or possibly in the future?

STEP 4: Your partner plays the "If it was my dream" game and shares their ideas, thoughts, and feelings about the dream, as if it had been theirs.

STEP 5: Summarize the dream in a pithy phrase, like a bumper sticker.

STEP 6: Identify what action steps you intend to take to honor your dream.

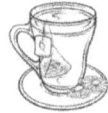 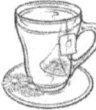

* Based on the work of Robert Moss.

WORKSHEET 9

Lightning Dreamwork

INSTRUCTIONS: Use the Lightning Dreamwork* framework to share dreams with others.

STEP 1: Explain your dream as clearly and simply as possible. Give it a title.

STEP 2: How did you feel upon awakening?

STEP 3: Reality check: Do you recognize anything from your life now or possibly in the future?

STEP 4: Your partner plays the "If it was my dream" game and shares their ideas, thoughts, and feelings about the dream, as if it had been theirs.

STEP 5: Summarize the dream in a pithy phrase, like a bumper sticker.

STEP 6: Identify what action steps you intend to take to honor your dream.

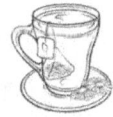 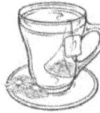

* Based on the work of Robert Moss.

WORKSHEET 9

Lightning Dreamwork

INSTRUCTIONS: Use the Lightning Dreamwork* framework to share dreams with others.

STEP 1: Explain your dream as clearly and simply as possible. Give it a title.

STEP 2: How did you feel upon awakening?

STEP 3: Reality check: Do you recognize anything from your life now or possibly in the future?

STEP 4: Your partner plays the "If it was my dream" game and shares their ideas, thoughts, and feelings about the dream, as if it had been theirs.

STEP 5: Summarize the dream in a pithy phrase, like a bumper sticker.

STEP 6: Identify what action steps you intend to take to honor your dream.

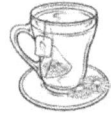 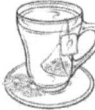

* Based on the work of Robert Moss.

WORKSHEET 9

Lightning Dreamwork

INSTRUCTIONS: Use the Lightning Dreamwork* framework to share dreams with others.

STEP 1: Explain your dream as clearly and simply as possible. Give it a title.

STEP 2: How did you feel upon awakening?

STEP 3: Reality check: Do you recognize anything from your life now or possibly in the future?

STEP 4: Your partner plays the "If it was my dream" game and shares their ideas, thoughts, and feelings about the dream, as if it had been theirs.

STEP 5: Summarize the dream in a pithy phrase, like a bumper sticker.

STEP 6: Identify what action steps you intend to take to honor your dream.

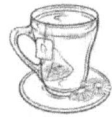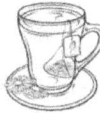

* Based on the work of Robert Moss.

WORKSHEET 9

Lightning Dreamwork

INSTRUCTIONS: Use the Lightning Dreamwork* framework to share dreams with others.

STEP 1: Explain your dream as clearly and simply as possible. Give it a title.

STEP 2: How did you feel upon awakening?

STEP 3: Reality check: Do you recognize anything from your life now or possibly in the future?

STEP 4: Your partner plays the "If it was my dream" game and shares their ideas, thoughts, and feelings about the dream, as if it had been theirs.

STEP 5: Summarize the dream in a pithy phrase, like a bumper sticker.

STEP 6: Identify what action steps you intend to take to honor your dream.

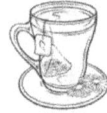 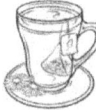

* Based on the work of Robert Moss.

WORKSHEET 10: HABIT TRACKER

What I Do to De-stress

WORKSHEET 10: HABIT TRACKER

What I Do to De-stress

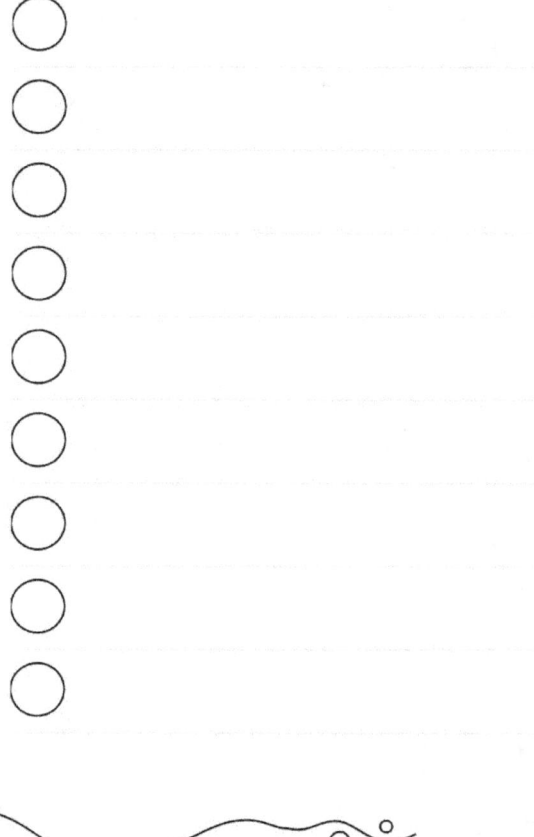

WORKSHEET 10: HABIT TRACKER

What I Do to De-stress

○

○

○

○

○

○

○

○

○

WORKSHEET 10: HABIT TRACKER

What I Do to De-stress

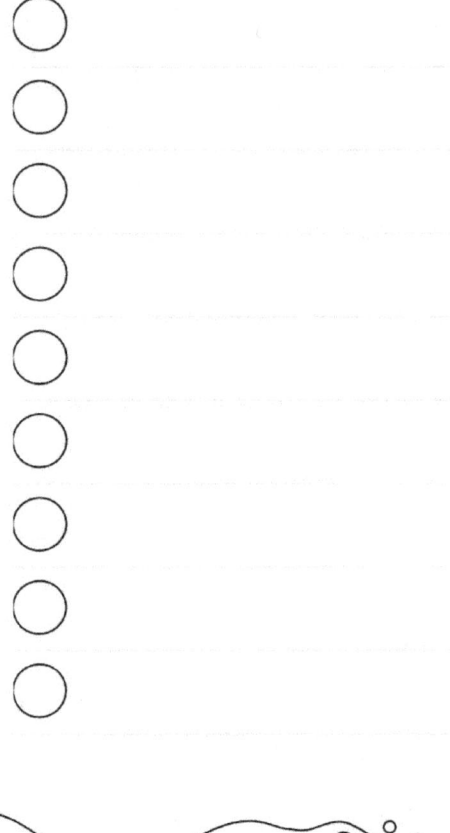

WORKSHEET 10: HABIT TRACKER

What I Do to De-stress

○

○

○

○

○

○

○

○

○

WORKSHEET 10: HABIT TRACKER

What I Do to De-stress

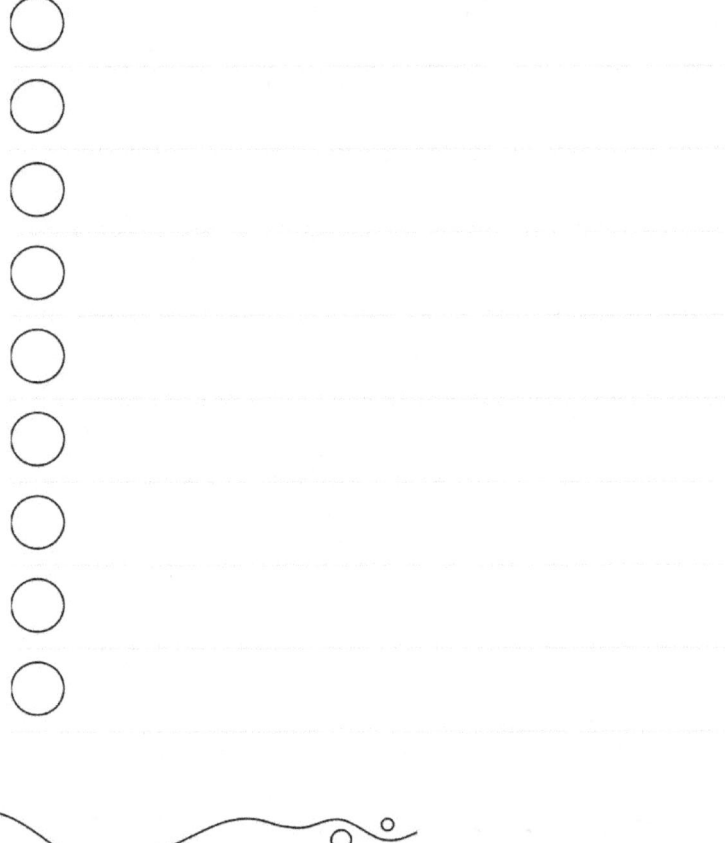

WORKSHEET 10: HABIT TRACKER

What I Do to De-stress

○

○

○

○

○

○

○

○

○

WORKSHEET 10: HABIT TRACKER

What I Do to De-stress

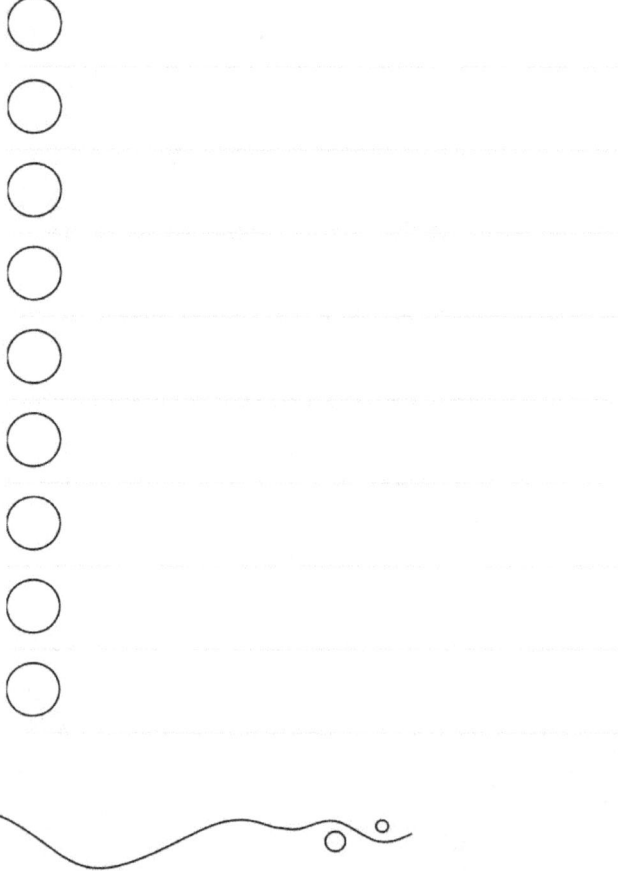

THE END

www.ingramcontent.com/pod-product-compliance
Lightning Source LLC
Chambersburg PA
CBHW071203120626
46546CB00006B/2390